UNDERSTANDING
PHOBIAS

by Maddie Spalding

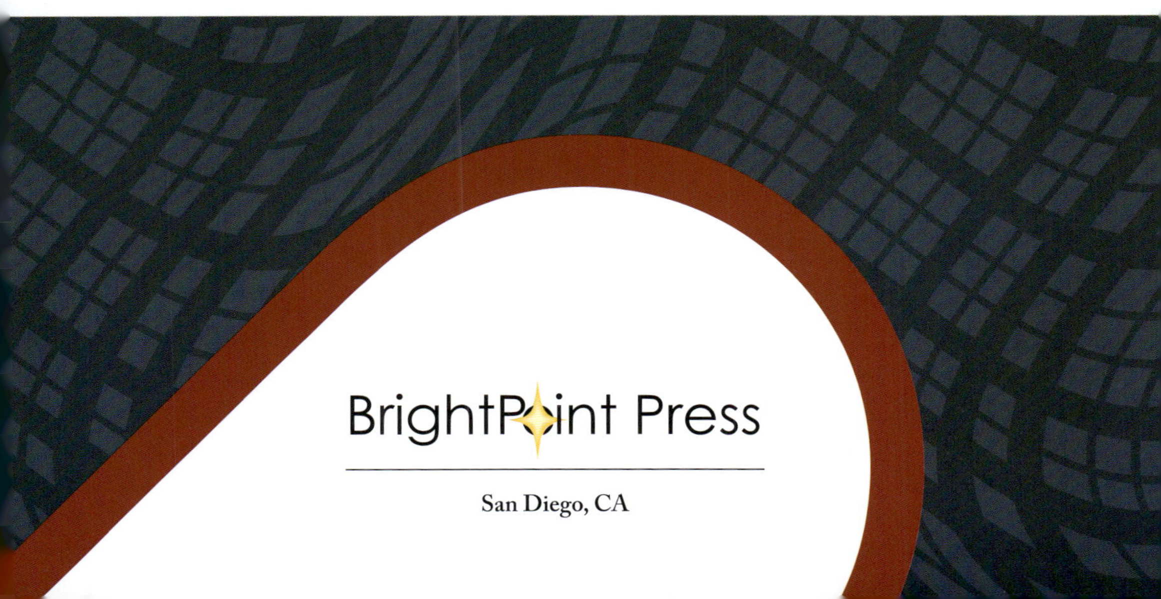

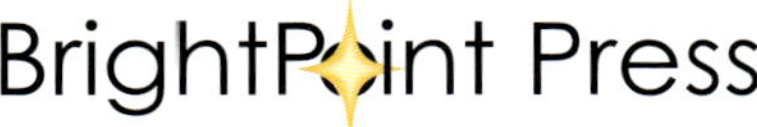

BrightPoint Press

Content Consultant: Christopher Bloom, PhD, Professor of Psychology, Providence College

LIBRARY OF CONGRESS CATALOGING-IN-PUBLICATION DATA

Names: Spalding, Maddie, author.
Title: Understanding phobias / by Maddie Spalding.
Description: San Diego, CA : BrightPoint Press, [2022] | Series: Mental health guides | Includes bibliographical references and index. | Audience: Grades 7-9
Identifiers: LCCN 2021009633 (print) | LCCN 2021009634 (eBook) | ISBN 9781678201401 (hardcover) | ISBN 9781678201418 (eBook)
Subjects: LCSH: Phobias--Juvenile literature. | Phobias--Treatment--Juvenile literature.
Classification: LCC RC535 .S638 2022 (print) | LCC RC535 (eBook) | DDC 616.85/225--dc23
LC record available at https:// ccn.loc.gov/2021009633
LC eBook record available at nttps://lccn.loc.gov/2021009634

CONTENTS

AT A GLANCE

- Phobias are intense fears of certain things or situations. These things or situations trigger a fear response. People with phobias avoid things that may trigger fear.

- A phobia is a type of anxiety disorder. People feel anxious when they think about triggers.

- There are three types of phobias. They are specific phobias, social anxiety disorder (SAD), and agoraphobia.

- Some people fear specific things such as needles. They have specific phobias. They may also fear specific situations. For example, they may fear enclosed spaces.

- People with SAD fear social situations. They worry that others will judge them.

- Phobias can affect people's work and social lives. They can also affect people's physical health.

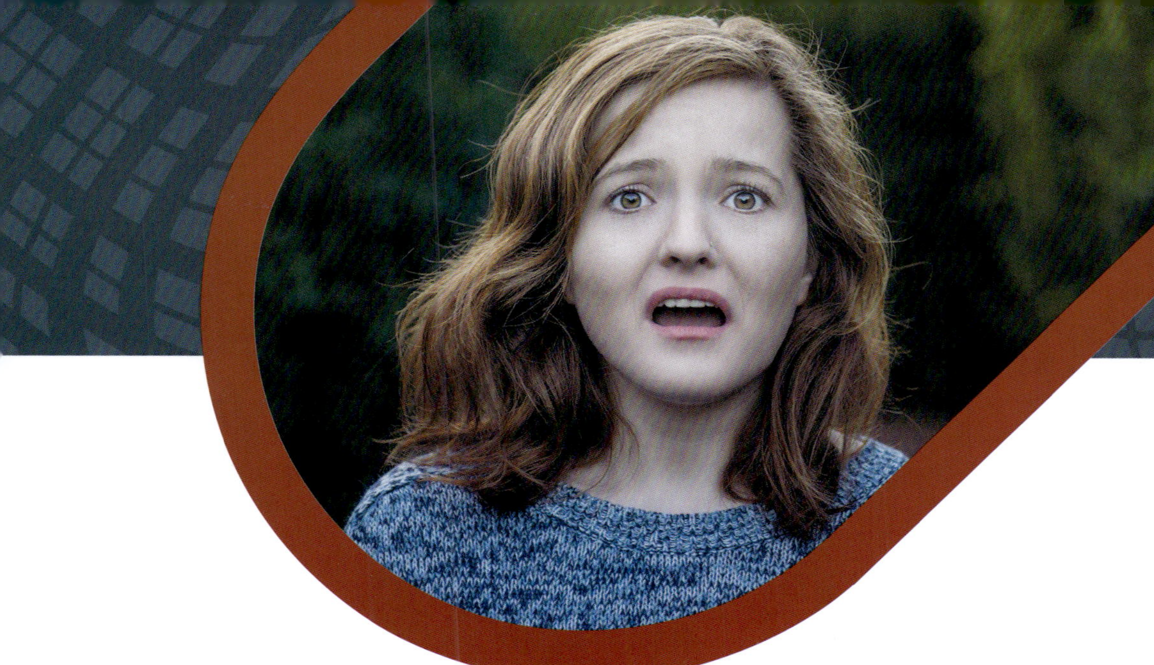

- People with agoraphobia fear places where escape is difficult. This could include places with crowds. It could also include public transportation.

- Phobias come with certain symptoms. These may include an increased heart rate. People may start to sweat or shake.

- Phobias are common. Approximately 13 percent of US adults develop phobias.

- Treatment can help people with phobias. Cognitive behavioral therapy (CBT) is often used to treat phobias.

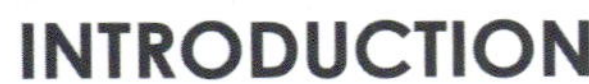

AIMEE'S STORY

Ten-year-old Aimee was stuck inside a cupboard. She had chosen to hide there during a game of hide-and-seek. But now she could not get out. The air felt warm. Aimee started to panic. She cried and screamed. She felt like she might die. People heard her and came to her rescue. They opened the cupboard door. Aimee had been inside the cupboard for only a

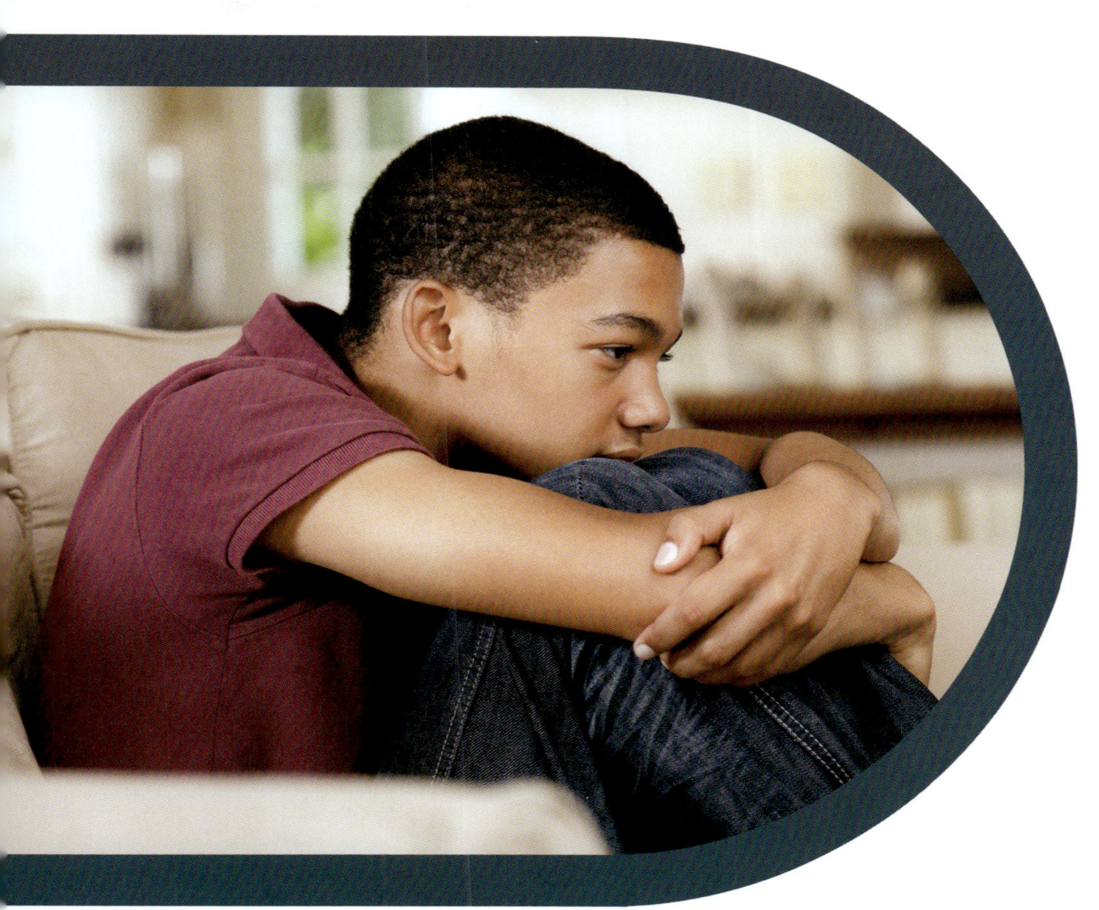

Phobias can cause extreme distress and anxiety.

few minutes. But to her, those minutes had

seemed like hours.

A couple of years later, Aimee was

eating lunch with friends. They were in a

classroom at school. The classroom door

got stuck. Aimee and her friends could not open it. The experience reminded Aimee of the time she had been trapped in the cupboard. She became frightened. She started to scream and cry. She had a panic attack. A panic attack is a feeling of intense discomfort or fear. A teacher heard Aimee and opened the door.

These experiences had lasting effects on Aimee. She began to check all doors and locks. She lived in fear of being trapped. She had developed claustrophobia. This is a fear of confined spaces. People with this phobia avoid these spaces. Aimee avoided

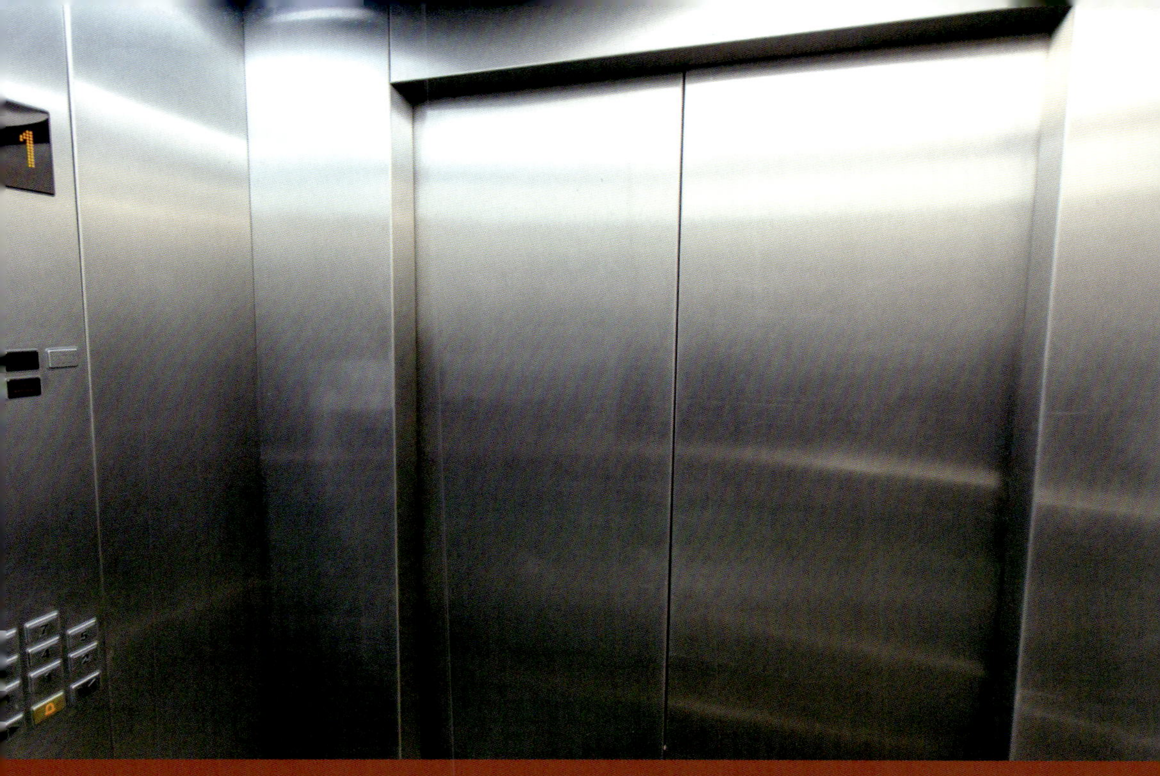

Someone with claustrophobia feels frightened in enclosed spaces such as elevators.

public restrooms, where she felt trapped.

She feared getting into taxis or cars with

automatic locks. She worked at a clothing

store as a teenager. But she could not

go into the changing rooms. Elevators

were Aimee's biggest fear. She panicked

whenever she saw elevator doors. Her fear
and anxiety affected her daily life.

FACING HER FEARS

Today, Aimee continues to encounter
challenges. But she has begun to face her
fears. She sees a therapist. Therapists are
trained professionals. They help people who
have mental health problems. The therapist
helps Aimee talk about her phobia. In 2017,
Aimee had a victory. She went on a plane
ride. She had avoided planes for a long
time. She thought she would feel trapped
on the plane. Aimee's therapist helped her
manage her fear.

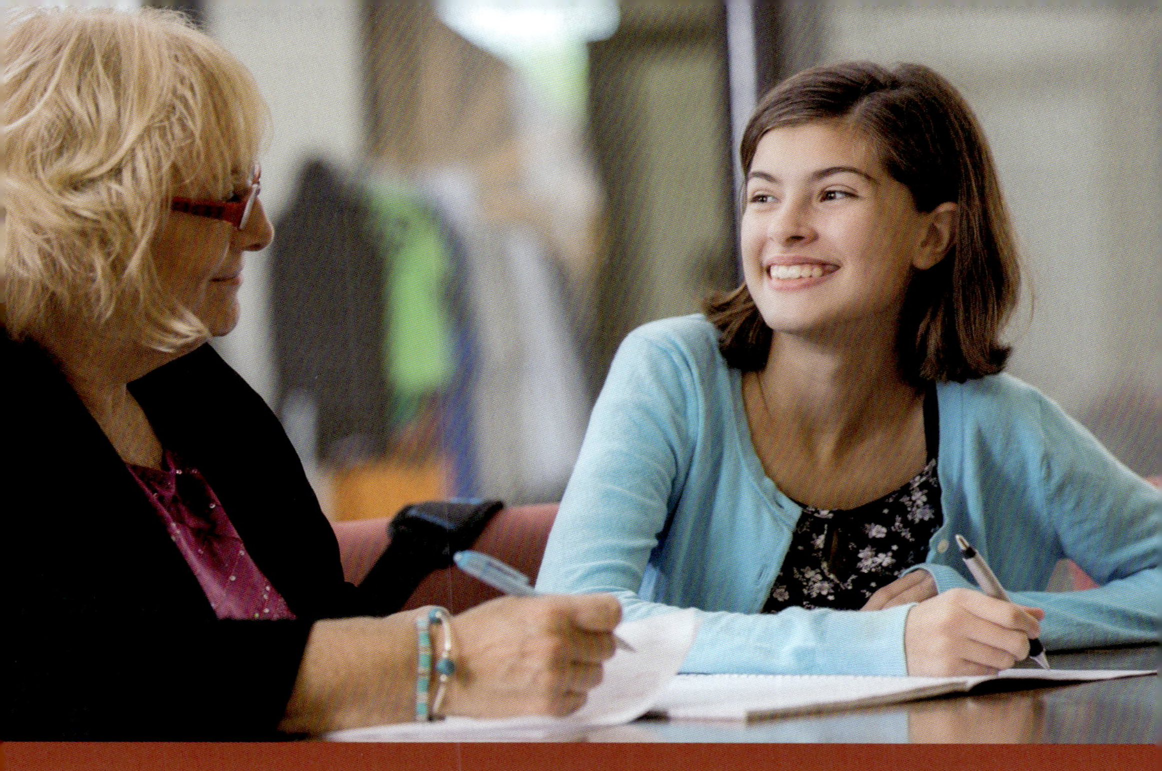

Therapy can help someone manage her phobia.

Aimee gained more self-confidence.
She went to college to study psychology.
She also started her own business. She
continues to achieve new goals. She has
hope for the future. Aimee's story shows
that it is possible for people to manage
their phobias.

WHAT ARE PHOBIAS?

Fear is a normal response to danger. A person's body releases **hormones**. These chemicals move through the bloodstream. The person's heart rate drops and then sharply increases. This sends more blood to the muscles and important organs. The person starts to breathe faster. Extra oxygen goes to the brain and makes

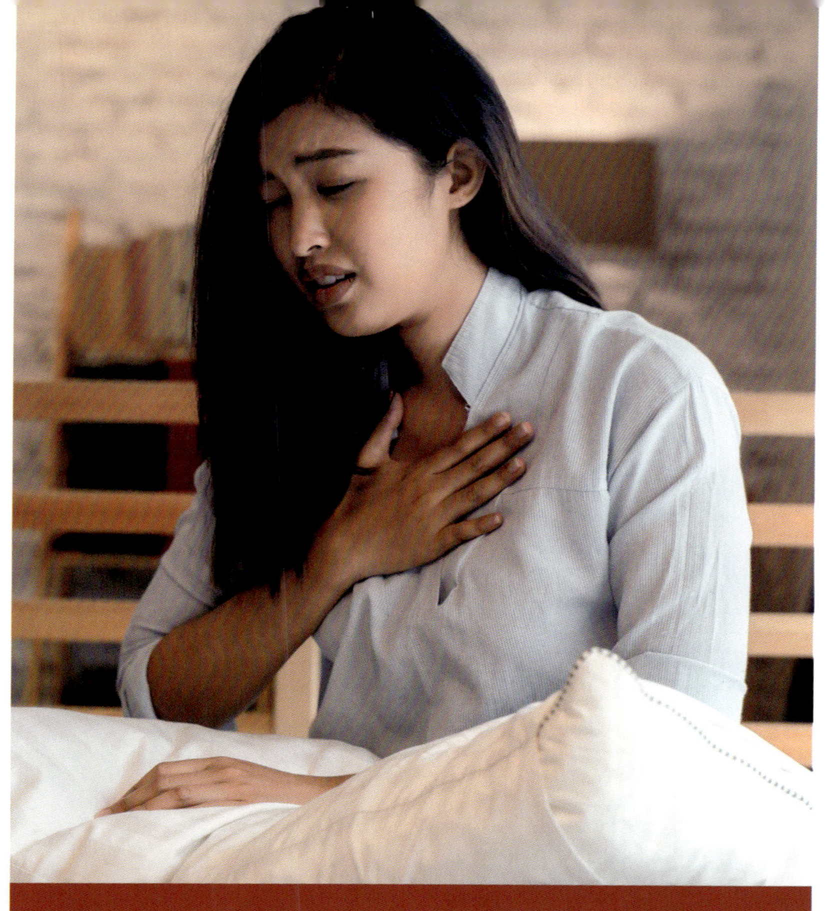

Fear causes a person's heart rate to increase.

the person more alert. Senses such as sight and hearing become sharper. The person becomes energized. All these things help someone react quickly. She may fight the threat. She may flee. Or she might freeze

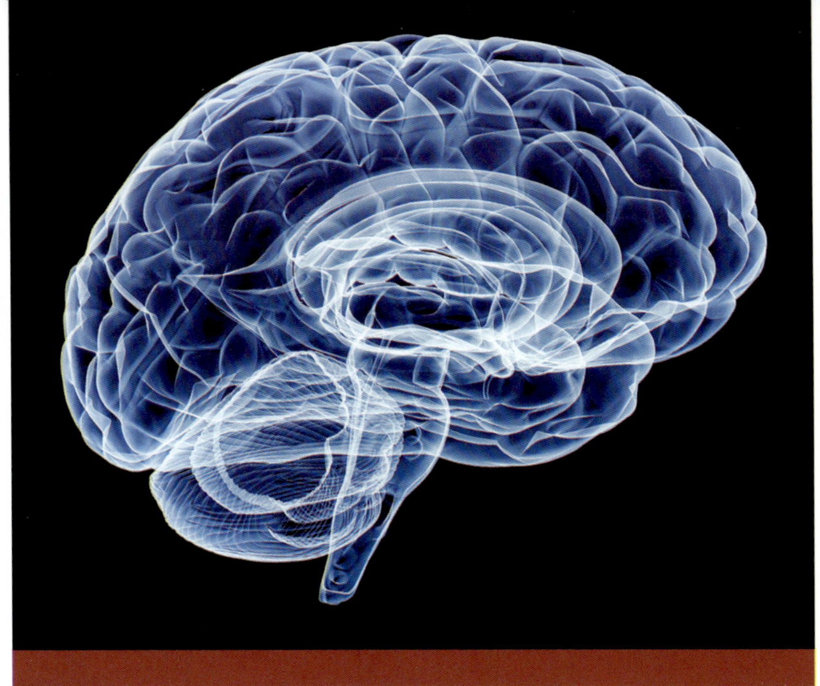

The brain becomes more alert during a fear response.

and do nothing. Her mind may go blank. She may feel numb. All fear responses start with freezing. Together these reactions are known as fight-flight-freeze responses. They help protect people from dangers.

Phobias often begin as a normal fear response. A person may face a real danger.

For example, Aimee was trapped in a cupboard. She felt intense fear. This fear became a phobia when it affected her daily life. A phobia is an unrealistic, persistent fear. She felt anxious when she thought about enclosed spaces. People with phobias think about potential threats. They avoid situations that they see as threatening. Aimee avoided crowds. She didn't take elevators. Anxiety took over her life. She found it hard to make friends. She explains, "People tend to think my experience is just a dislike. What they don't understand is the absolute fear."[1]

TYPES OF PHOBIAS

A phobia is a type of anxiety disorder.
Anxiety disorders are the most common
type of mental illness in the United States.
These disorders may disrupt everyday
life. They can change people's thoughts
and moods. They can also affect people's
physical health.

There are three main types of phobias.
One type is specific phobias. People with
specific phobias may fear certain objects or
animals. Fear of needles and fear of spiders
are common. A person might have a
specific phobia of heights. Certain situations

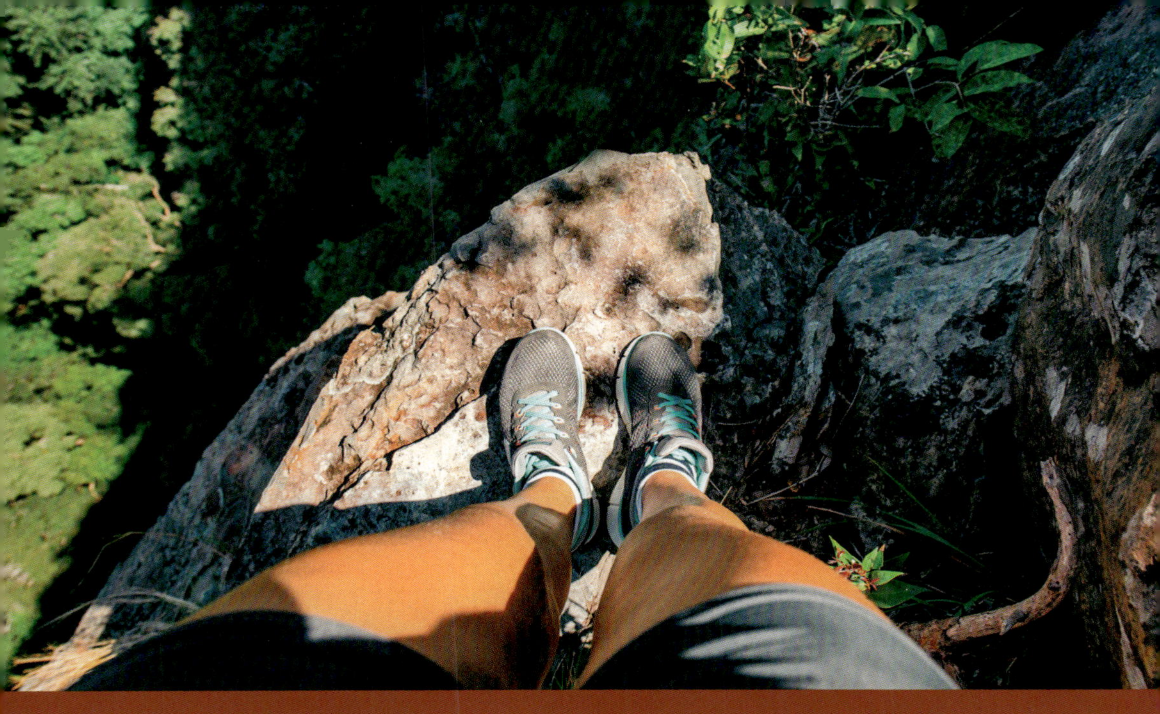

Fear of heights is a common phobia.

could cause fear too. These might include

being on an elevator. Some people fear

going to the doctor. Claustrophobia

is a specific phobia. Fear of blood is

another example.

Social anxiety disorder (SAD) is another

type of phobia. It is also known as social

phobia. It involves a fear of social situations.
These situations might include meeting
new people. Performance situations can
cause anxiety too. Some people may fear
public speaking. Others may fear being
watched. They may avoid eating or drinking

MULTIPLE PHOBIAS

Most people with a specific phobia diagnosis
have multiple fears. On average, they have
three specific phobias. For example, they
might fear storms, flying, and enclosed spaces.
These fears may relate to each other. Someone
may be afraid of flying because an airplane is
an enclosed space. The fear may come from
a certain event. The event often happens in
childhood. But it may also happen later in life.

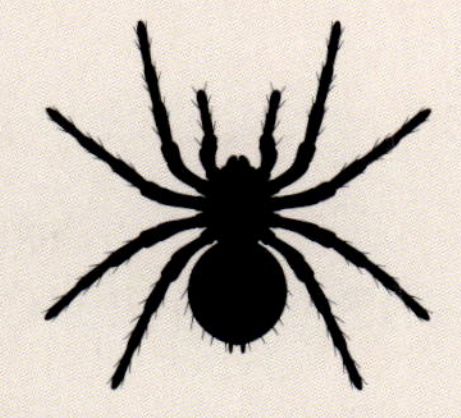

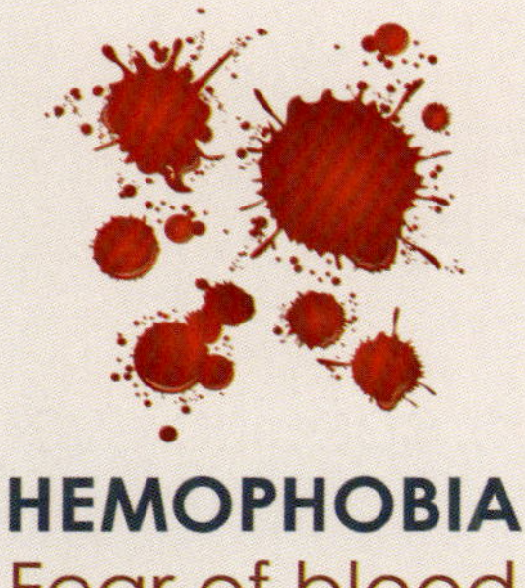

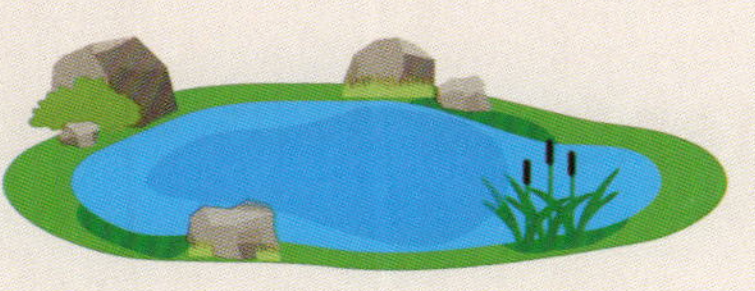

Each specific phobia has a unique name. This chart names some of the common specific phobias.

around others. They worry that people will judge them.

The third type of phobia is agoraphobia. People with agoraphobia fear places where it would be difficult to escape.

These are often public places. People with this phobia might avoid crowds or public transportation. They have extreme anxiety in these situations.

TRAUMA AND EXPERIENCES

A phobia often arises from a specific event. The event may have been traumatic. A traumatic event causes a strong emotional response. People may be in shock after the event. They might avoid objects or situations related to the event. For example, an animal attack can be traumatic. The person who was attacked might develop an animal phobia. Someone who had a

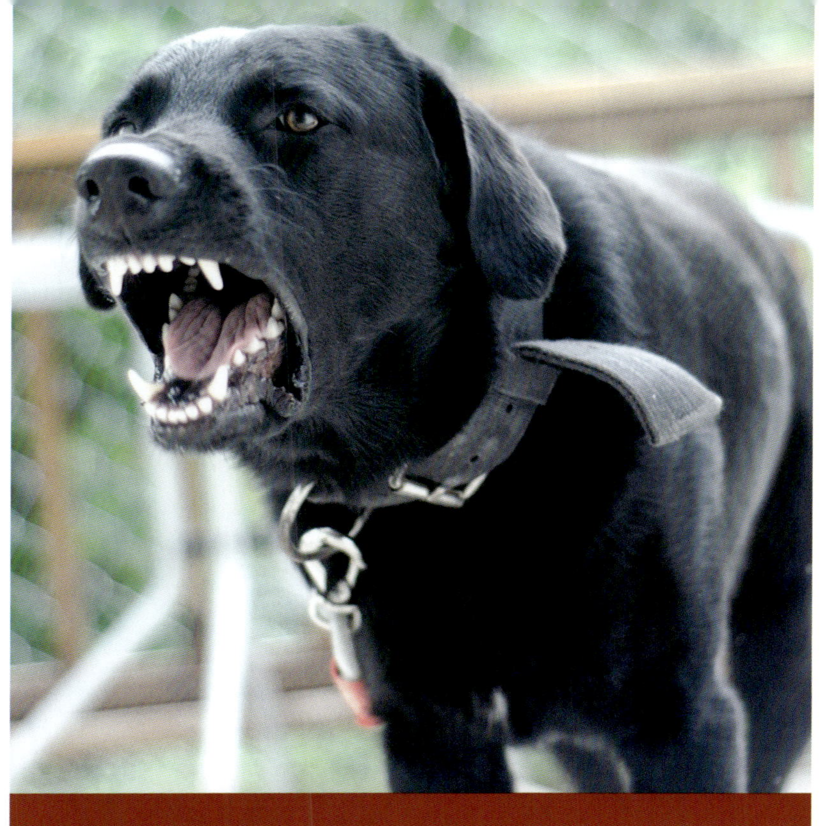

Someone who has been attacked by a dog may develop a phobia of dogs.

near-drowning experience could develop a

water phobia.

Stacey Griffith almost drowned while

surfing in the ocean. A strong current

pulled her away from the shore. It pushed

her underwater. She struggled to breathe.

A lifeguard saved her. Griffith was an experienced swimmer. She was a lifeguard herself. But she developed a water phobia after this experience. She says, "I was terrified to get back in the water. It took me

DIAGNOSING PHOBIAS

Therapists need to diagnose a disorder in order to treat it. They look at a person's **symptoms**. They see if these symptoms match a certain disorder. They use the *Diagnostic and Statistical Manual of Mental Disorders* (*DSM*). The *DSM* lists all types of mental disorders. It explains their symptoms. Experts regularly update the *DSM*. The most recent version in 2020 was the *DSM-5*.

five years before I even dipped a toe in the ocean again."[2]

Some people may not experience a frightening event firsthand. They may see another person react strongly to an event or situation. They might then develop a phobia of the event or situation. Sometimes people develop phobias after learning about an event. For example, someone might hear about a plane crash. The person might develop a phobia of planes. Dr. Craig April treats people who have anxiety disorders. He says, "One can develop a phobia simply through observation and learning."[3]

GENES AND ENVIRONMENT

Studies show that phobias may run in families. If a child's parent has a phobia, the child may be more likely to develop that phobia. Some researchers have studied twins. They found that twins are likely to share phobias. When one twin had a specific phobia, the other had a 30 percent chance of having the same fear. With agoraphobia, the chance was 39 percent.

Blood and medical phobias are more likely to run in families. Agata Boxe is a writer and editor. Boxe and her sister have needle phobias. Their mother has a medical

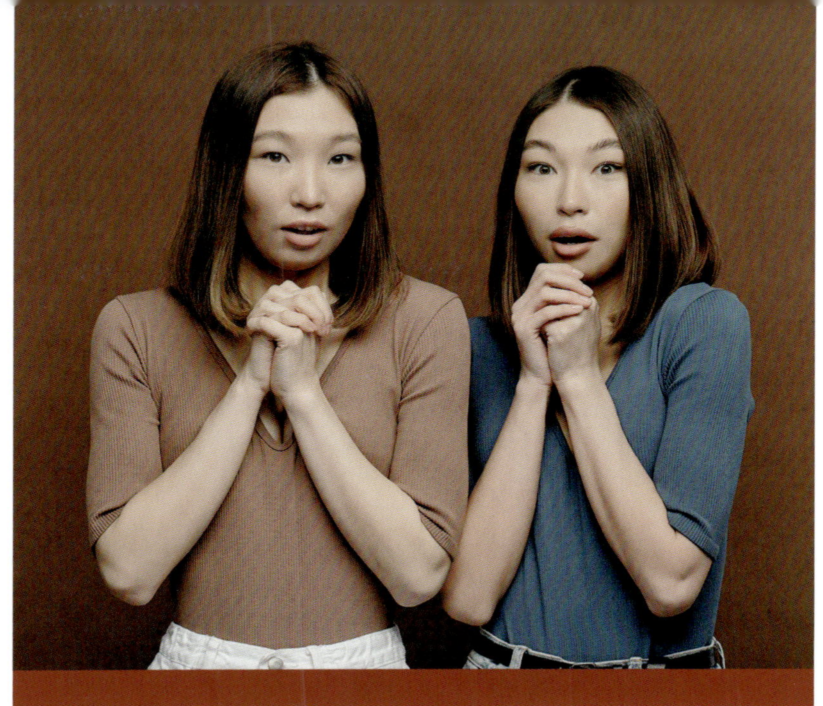

Studies show that twins may share the same phobia.

phobia. Boxe's phobia started in childhood.

She says, "Even thinking about [needles]

sends me spiraling."[4] She sometimes faints

around needles.

Certain phobias are more likely to

be caused by a person's experiences.

For example, someone with claustrophobia

might have had a bad experience. He might have been stuck in an elevator before.

A combination of factors makes it more likely for some people to develop phobias. Some people with phobias have had a bad experience that caused the fear. They may also have relatives with phobias. Their environment and **genes** both play a role. For example, a child's parent might have a needle phobia. The child may have genes that make it more likely he will develop a phobia. The parent might be anxious when the child gets a shot. The child may learn to be afraid of needles because of

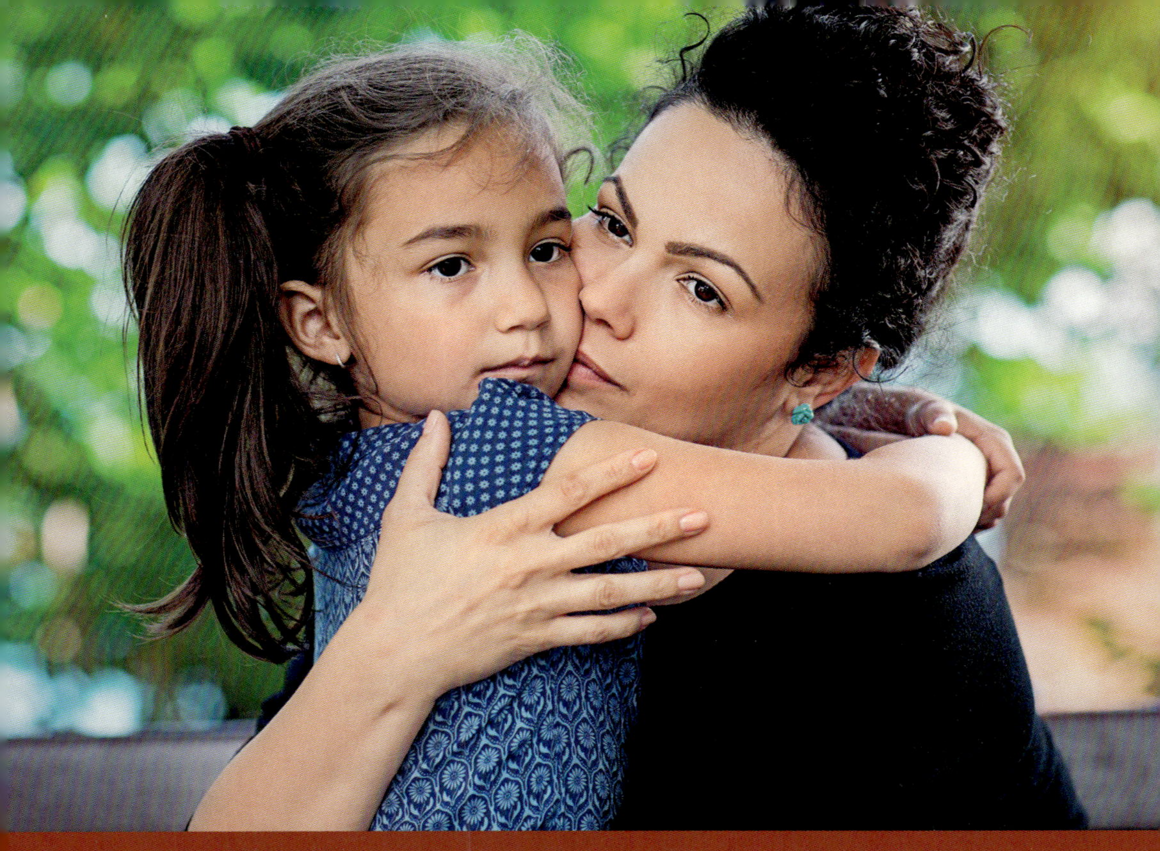

A child may learn to fear certain objects from her parent's reaction.

the parent's reaction. The parent may

repeatedly tell the child, "It's OK." He says

this to comfort the child. But experts have

found that this communicates anxiety. It can

make the child more distressed.

CHAPTER TWO

HOW DO PHOBIAS AFFECT PEOPLE?

Phobias cause fear that is more intense than normal fear responses. People with phobias experience a strong sense of danger. This feeling of danger is greater than the actual threat. People may spend a lot of time thinking about their fears. These thoughts may cause distress. People may

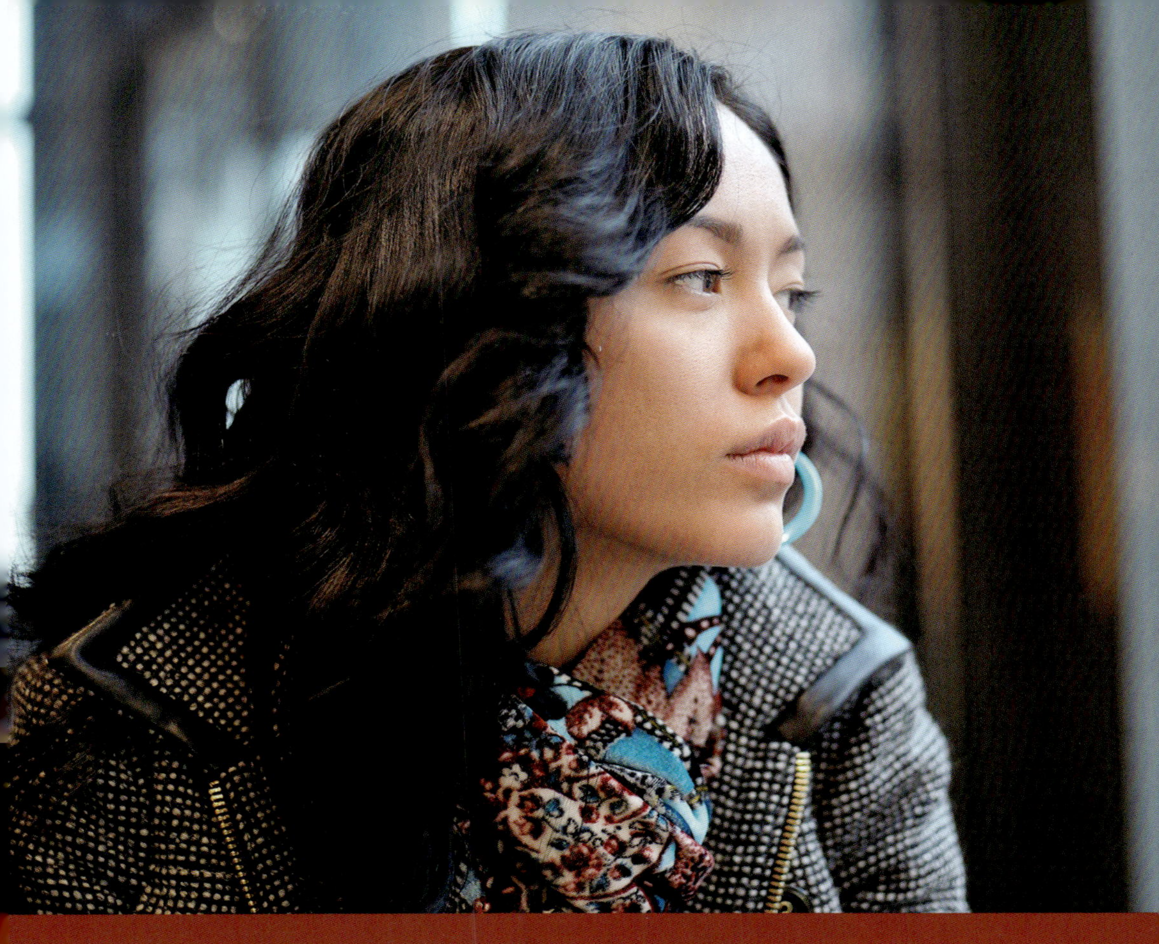

go out of their way to avoid feared objects

or situations. These objects or situations

trigger fear responses. Therapists look for

these signs when they diagnose phobias.

People usually experience the strong fear response to the object or situation for six months or more.

Phobias also cause anxiety. The body reacts to anxiety. A person's heart rate increases when he feels anxious. His **blood pressure** goes up. He might start sweating or shaking.

Physical symptoms can be different with a blood or medical phobia. First a person's heart rate increases. Then it drops. The person's blood pressure drops too. This sudden drop in blood pressure makes him feel light-headed. He might faint.

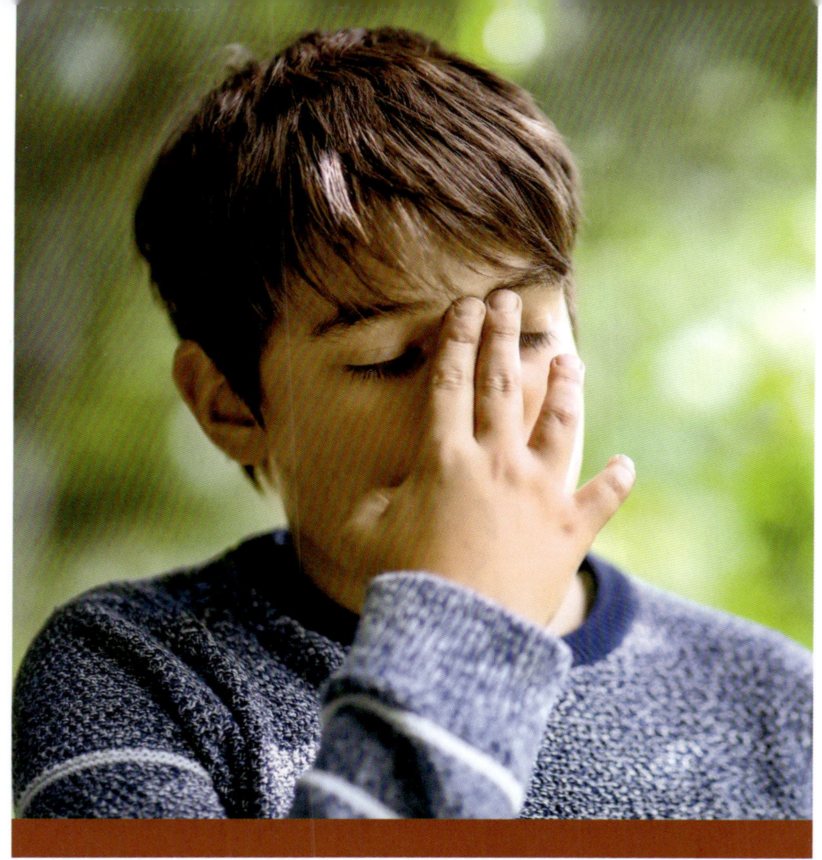

Seeing blood may cause someone with a medical phobia to feel light-headed and faint.

Nearly 70 percent of people with this phobia faint in medical situations.

PANIC ATTACKS

Some people with phobias have panic attacks. Panic is an extreme form of anxiety.

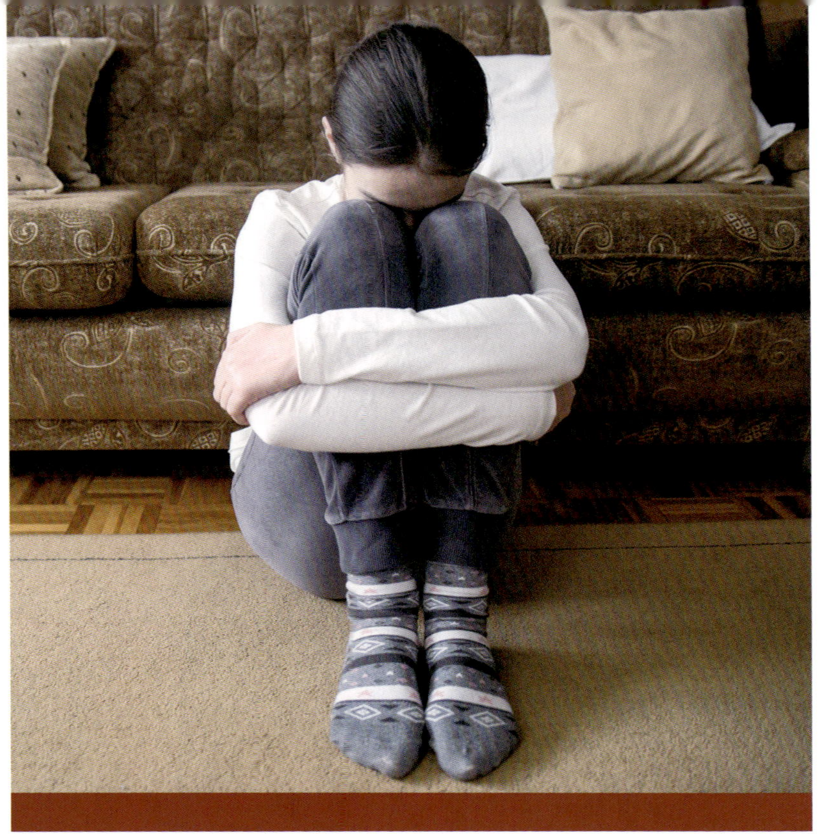

Phobias may cause panic attacks.

A panic attack is an intense feeling of fear or discomfort.

A panic attack causes a fight-flight-freeze response. The attack occurs suddenly. It may happen when a person sees a trigger. Even thinking about a trigger can

cause a panic attack. A panic attack
causes a person's heart to race. The
person could have difficulty breathing. She
may feel as if she is choking. She might
have chest pain or feel dizzy or nauseous.
She could feel hot or cold. Other symptoms
include feeling numb. The person may
feel tingling in her body. She may have an
out-of-body experience. She might feel like
she will lose control.

A panic attack usually lasts between five
and twenty minutes. These attacks are not
dangerous. They do not cause permanent
harm. But they can be scary. Marie is a

woman with agoraphobia. She also has
had panic attacks. She wrote about her
experience for a mental health website.
Marie says, "I had labored, heavy breathing.
I . . . kept thinking that I would freak out
or die."[5]

PANIC DISORDER

Some people have recurring panic attacks.
These people might have panic disorder (PD).
PD is not a phobia. But it is a type of anxiety
disorder. PD affects a person's thoughts and
behaviors. The panic attacks are unexpected.
The person worries about when the next attack
will happen. He may believe he will lose control.
He might avoid unfamiliar situations. These
thoughts and behaviors must last a month to be
diagnosed as PD.

Many people with agoraphobia have panic attacks. They may have had a panic attack in a public place before. Then they start to avoid public places. People might fear that they won't be able to escape if they have a panic attack. They might also fear that they won't be able to find help.

DAILY LIFE WITH A PHOBIA

In some cases, phobias do not interfere with people's everyday lives. For example, some people have a phobia of cats. This may not affect them much if they do not see cats often. But many people have phobias of common situations or objects. They try to avoid these triggers. This can affect their home, work, and social lives.

People with SAD avoid social situations. They may have difficulty making friends. They may isolate themselves. This can affect their relationships. It can also affect their schooling and employment. Children with SAD may fear social interactions at school. They might try to avoid going to school. Adults with SAD might find job interviews challenging.

Phobias cause extreme anxiety. This can affect people's performance at school or work. People may not be able

to concentrate well. They may not be able
to remember information. Their grades or
careers might suffer.

Agoraphobia limits how people travel. It
also affects the types of places they choose

POST-TRAUMATIC STRESS DISORDER

Some people go through events that cause
trauma. For example, they might experience
a car crash. They could develop a driving
phobia. They could also develop post-traumatic
stress disorder (PTSD). People with PTSD have
strong responses to triggers. They might have
flashbacks. Flashbacks happen when people
relive the event. People with PTSD may have
difficulty sleeping. They may startle easily. They
might have out-of-body experiences. PTSD
affects people's thoughts too. People may find
it hard to trust others.

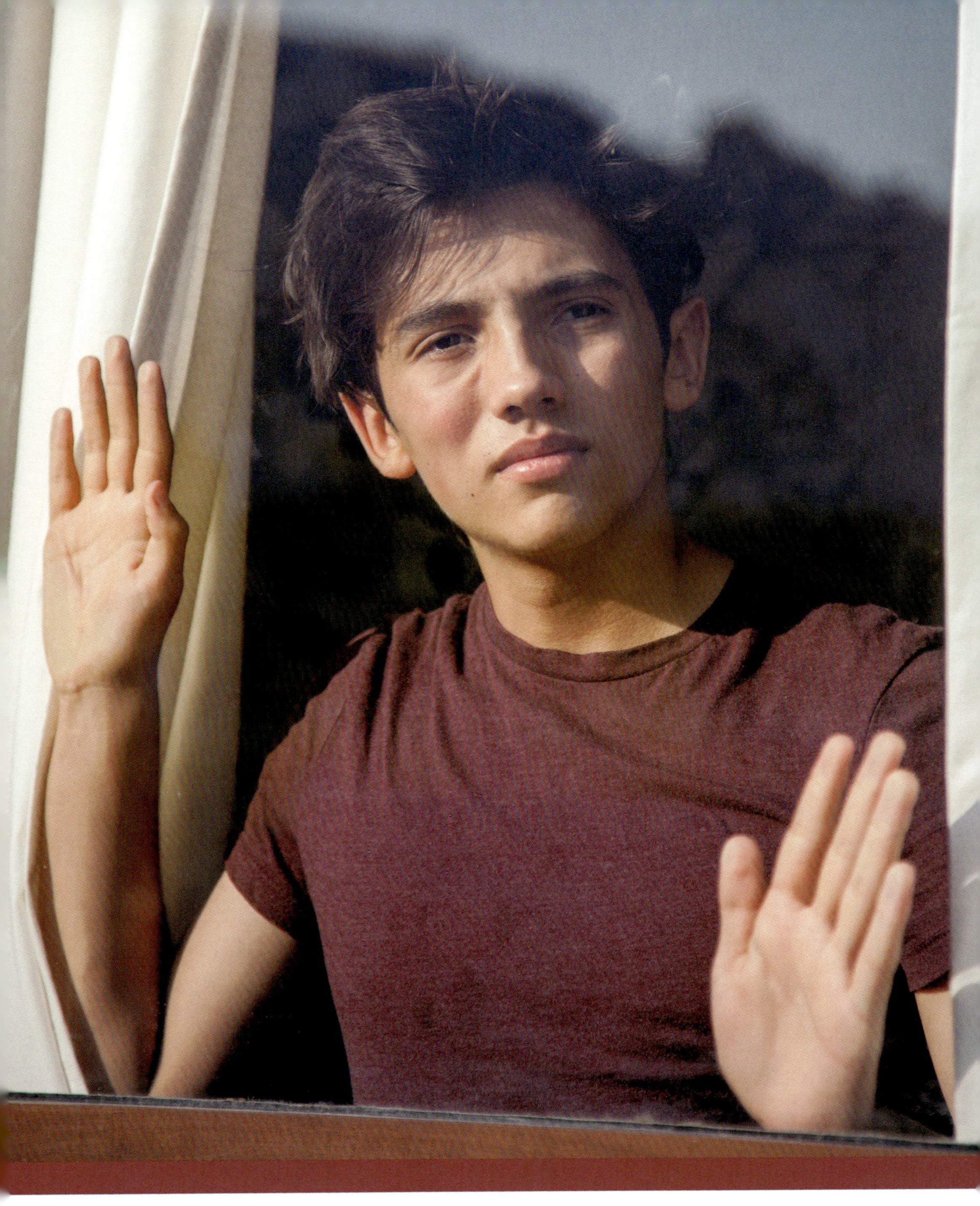

Someone with agoraphobia may avoid going outside.

to go to. People with agoraphobia may avoid public transportation. They might fear going into stores. They might even fear leaving their homes alone. In extreme cases, people may stop going outside. They may stop going to work. They may have people bring groceries to their homes. They rely on others to meet their needs. This can put a strain on their relationships. It can also affect their health. They may be afraid to leave their homes to go to the doctor.

LIVING WITH A SPECIFIC PHOBIA

Specific phobias can affect people's lives in many ways too. People with needle or medical phobias may stop going to the doctor or dentist. Their health may worsen as a result. Keith Lamb has a needle phobia. He says, "I am pain sensitive. I don't faint. I just get really scared."[6] He shakes and sweats. At one point, Lamb had an infection in his teeth and gums. The infection was life-threatening. But he avoided going to the dentist for months.

People might come across triggers while at home, school, or work. For example, a child may have a phobia of bugs. He might stop going outside during recess. Someone with claustrophobia might avoid elevators.

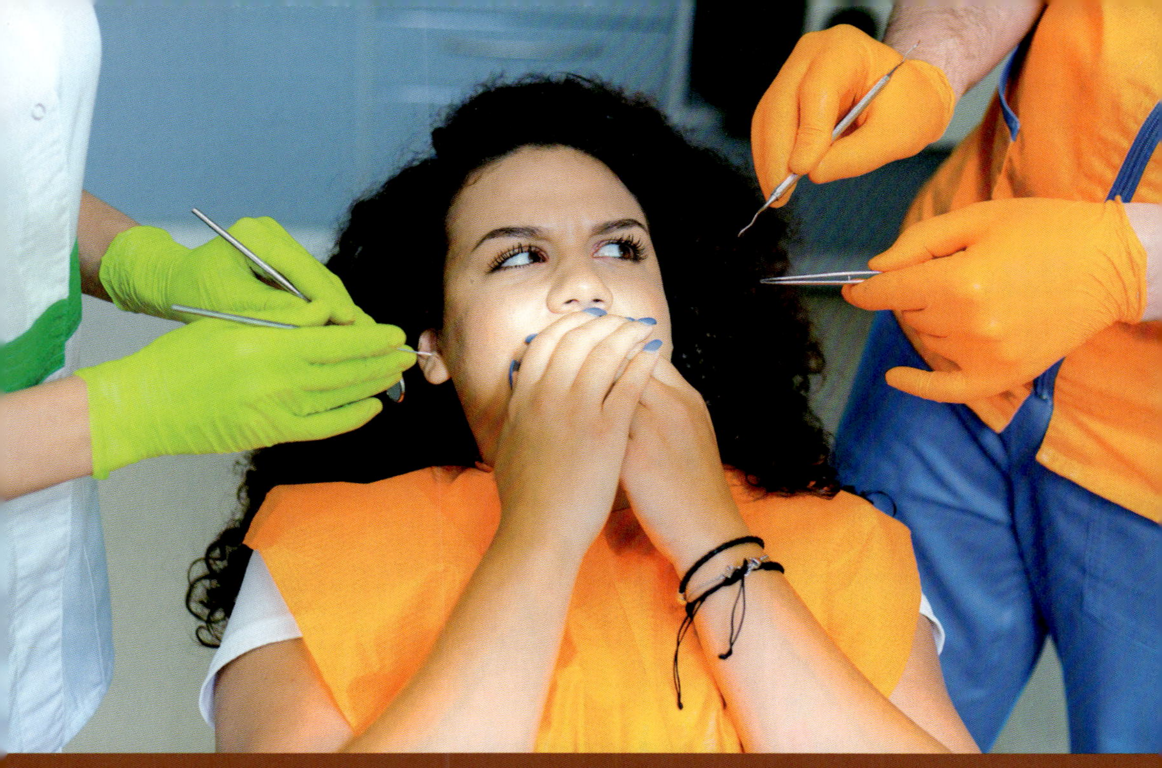

A dental phobia may cause someone to stop going to the dentist.

She may work in a tall office building.

She may have to walk up the stairs every

day. Phobias can also affect people's

employment. A job promotion may require

plane travel. Someone with a fear of planes

might pass up the promotion.

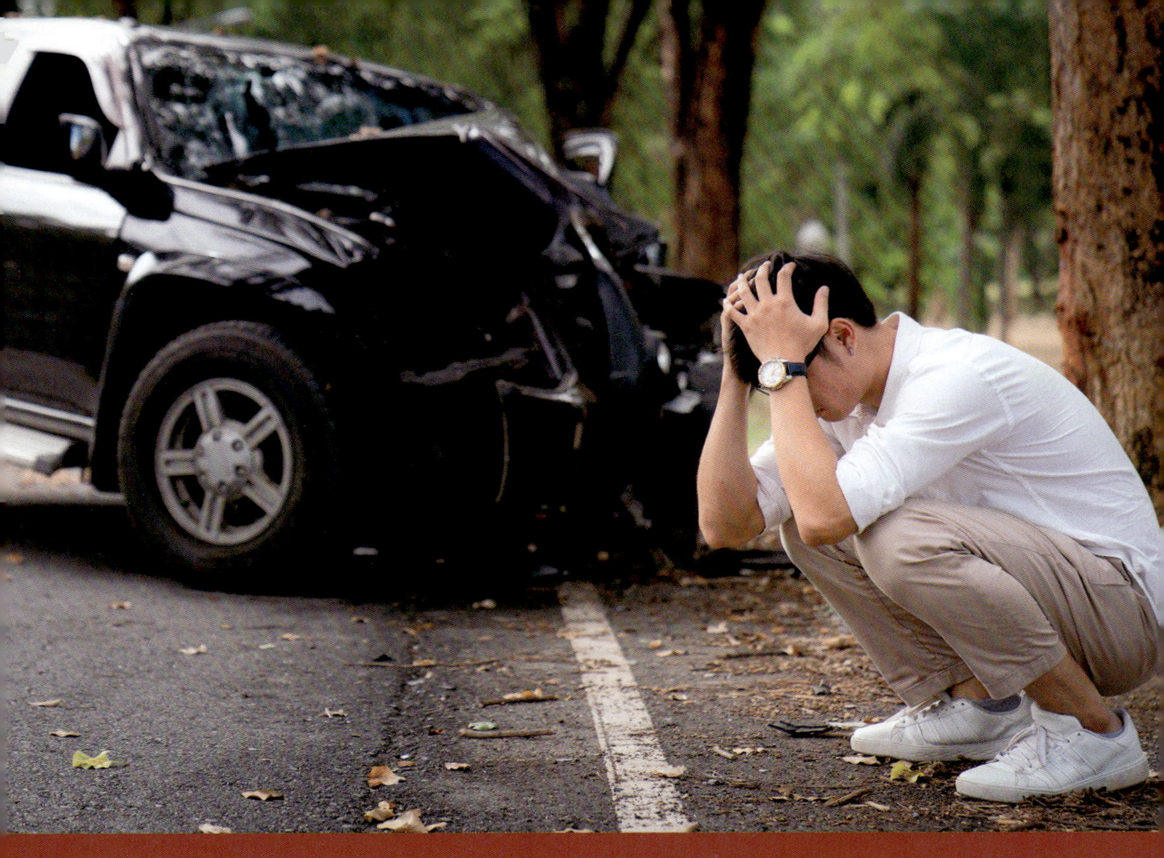

A car accident may cause a driving phobia to develop.

Some phobias interfere with people's ability to travel. Many people have driving phobias. They may have gotten into a car accident. Or they may have a history of panic attacks. They might fear that they will have a panic attack while driving. There are many reasons why phobias develop.

Phobias can affect people's travel routes too. For example, the fastest route to a person's workplace may be over a high bridge. If she has a phobia of heights, she may change her route to avoid the bridge. Then it will take her longer to get to work. Phobias can change people's lives in all these ways and more.

CHAPTER THREE

HOW DO PHOBIAS AFFECT SOCIETY?

Phobias affect both individuals and society as a whole. Phobias can arise at any age. Some people develop phobias in childhood. Others develop phobias as teens or adults.

HOW COMMON ARE PHOBIAS?

Approximately 13 percent of US adults develop phobias. Five percent of

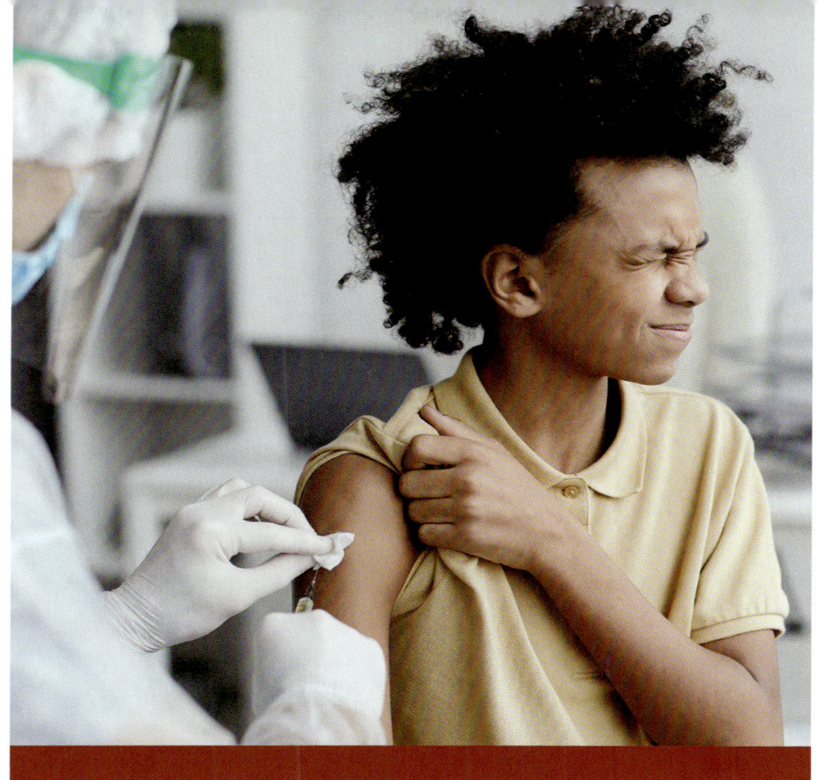

Phobias can develop at any age.

US children have specific phobias.

Childhood specific phobias usually start between five and nine years old. Some fears are common. They may not be phobias. Infants often fear loud noises and strangers. Young children may fear the dark. They also may fear imaginary beings such as monsters. These fears are phobias if they affect the child's functioning. Children may express their fears differently than adults. Children may cry or throw tantrums.

Childhood specific phobias may last only a short time. They may fade as people age. Teens are the most likely age group to

MULTIPLE DISORDERS

People with phobias are more likely to have other mental health disorders. These include other anxiety disorders. They also include depression. Depression is a feeling of sadness. It can cause a loss of interest in activities. People with phobias are also at risk of developing substance use disorders. They may become addicted to drugs or alcohol.

develop specific phobias. Specific phobias affect 16 percent of US teens. They affect about 5 percent of US adults.

SAD is also prevalent in the United States. Teens are most likely to develop SAD. Sixteen percent of US teens are diagnosed with SAD. The rate is 12 percent for US adults. Children are the least likely age group to be diagnosed with SAD. Five percent of US children are diagnosed with SAD. But symptoms often begin in childhood. For example, children may cry or refuse to speak in social situations.

Most people develop SAD between eight
and fifteen years old.

Nearly 2 percent of the US population
has agoraphobia. Children can develop
this phobia. But it is more common among
teens and adults. The average age when
people first notice symptoms is seventeen
years old.

Anxiety is more common among women
than men. Women are twice as likely as
men to develop most types of phobias. The
exception is blood and medical phobias.
Both genders are equally likely to have
these phobias.

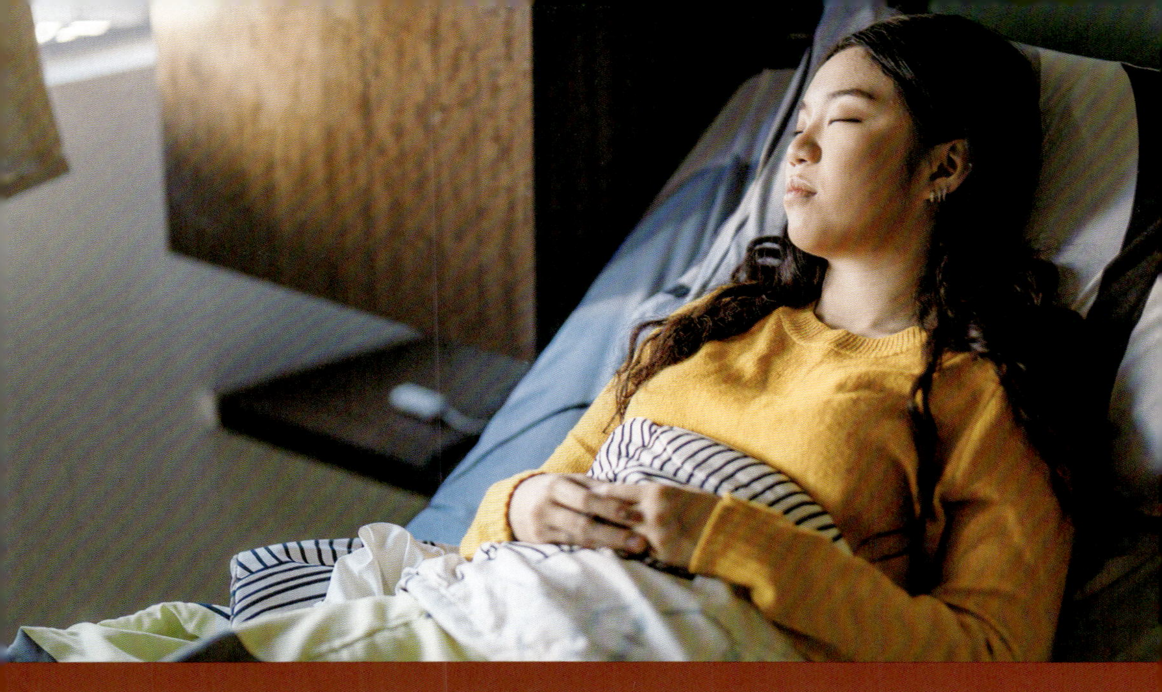

HEALTH CARE

Phobias can affect society in many ways. People with phobias may not access health care when needed. Those with agoraphobia may not want to leave their homes. Those who have blood or medical phobias fear going to the doctor.

People might feel embarrassed by their phobias. They may experience **stigma**. Other people might not understand the disorder. They may think that someone should be able to overcome a phobia by himself. They may believe that someone with a phobia is exaggerating his fear. This can cause a person with a phobia to feel ashamed. But having a mental illness is not shameful.

Feelings of shame can prevent people with phobias from seeking help. They may delay getting treatment. This can have serious consequences. People with phobias

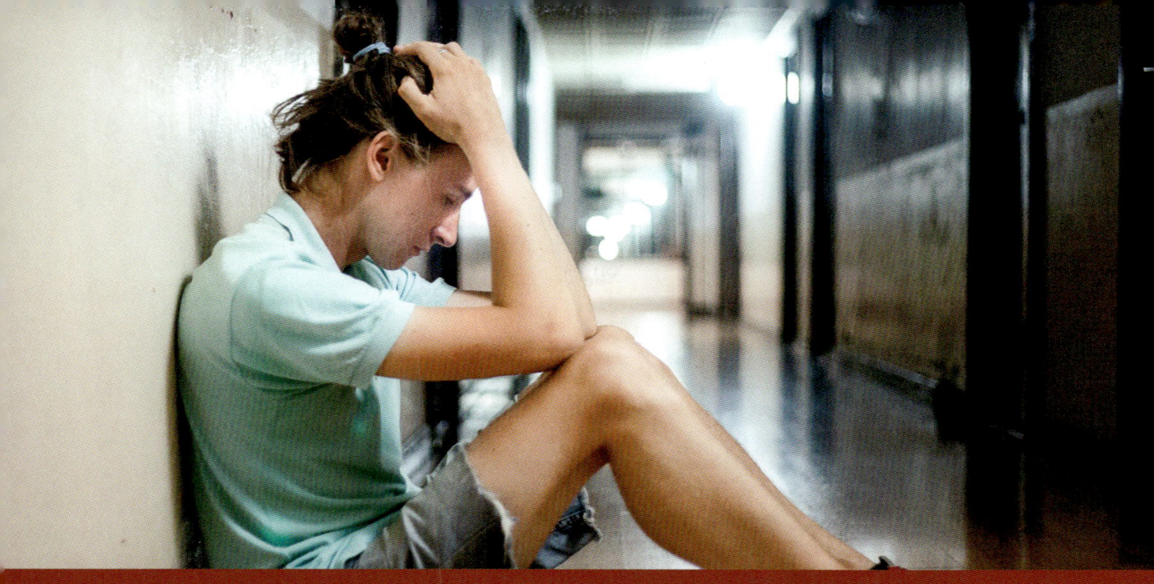

may stop telling others about their feelings.

Their relationships may suffer. They may

feel isolated due to lack of support from

family and friends. People with phobias may

also develop life-threatening conditions.

They might have to pay more for health care

if their health worsens. Dr. Bruce Peltier

is a psychology professor. He works with

people who have dental phobias. He says,
"A lot of their fears stem from the perceived
lack of control."[7] He suggests that dentists
allow these patients to ask for breaks. This
gives control back to the patients.

Some people need to give themselves
daily injections to manage medical
conditions. People with a needle phobia
might refuse these treatments. This could
be deadly.

They might also avoid vaccines. Vaccines
are usually given as shots. They protect
people from diseases. People who do
not get these shots are not protected.

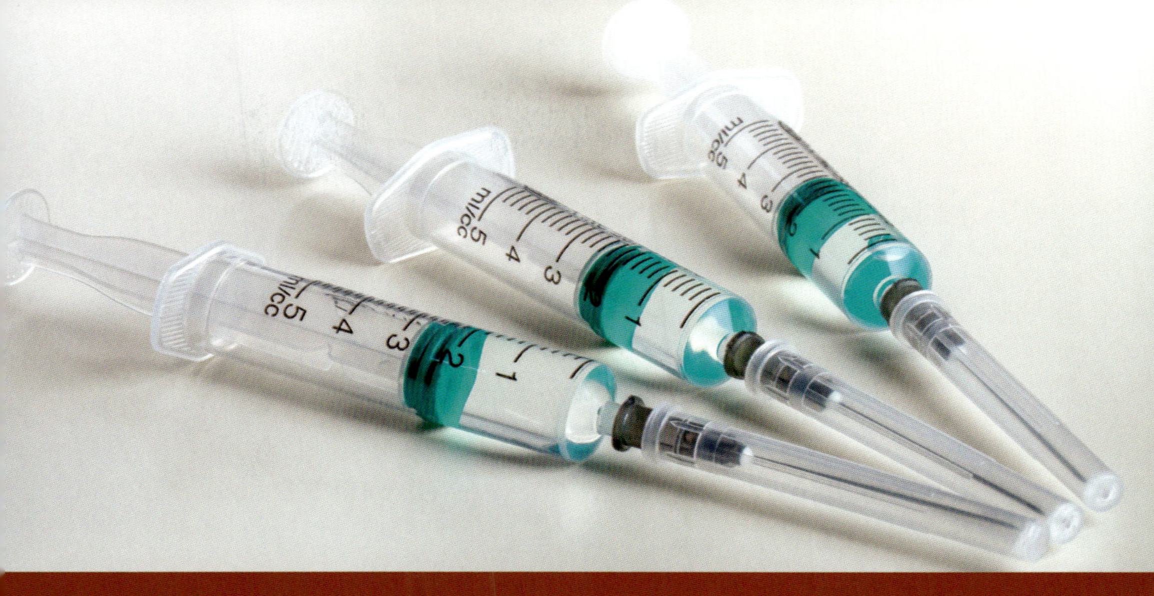

Fear of needles is a common phobia.

They might get sick. They could spread disease to other people.

EMPLOYMENT

Phobias may also affect people's employment. The phobia could take over their lives. People may find it hard to focus while at work. Phobias can also limit people's job options. One study looked at

how SAD affected people's careers. About
20 percent of people with SAD turned down
new jobs because they involved more social
interaction. People with SAD are more likely
to be unemployed than those without SAD.
Other phobias can cause unemployment
too. People with severe phobias may not
leave their homes often.

Keith Lamb's needle phobia almost cost
him his career. Lamb is an emergency
medical technician (EMT). EMTs provide
care to people in emergencies. He
sometimes has to inject patients. He
learned how to do this during EMT training.

He had to pair up with someone. They were told to practice injecting each other. Lamb does not mind using needles on others. But he fears getting injections. He told this to his instructor. The instructor did not understand at first. He told Lamb the exercise was required. Lamb explained his phobia. Finally, the instructor changed his mind. Lamb did not have to be injected. He passed the class and became an EMT. Lamb thinks his needle phobia gives him an advantage. It helps him sympathize with his patients. He says, "I am extremely sensitive to the patient's pain."[8]

In some cases, phobias can cause disability. A disability is a condition that limits someone's ability to do important activities. For example, a person might be unable to work or travel. The phobia interferes with her everyday life. People with phobias that cause disability may be able

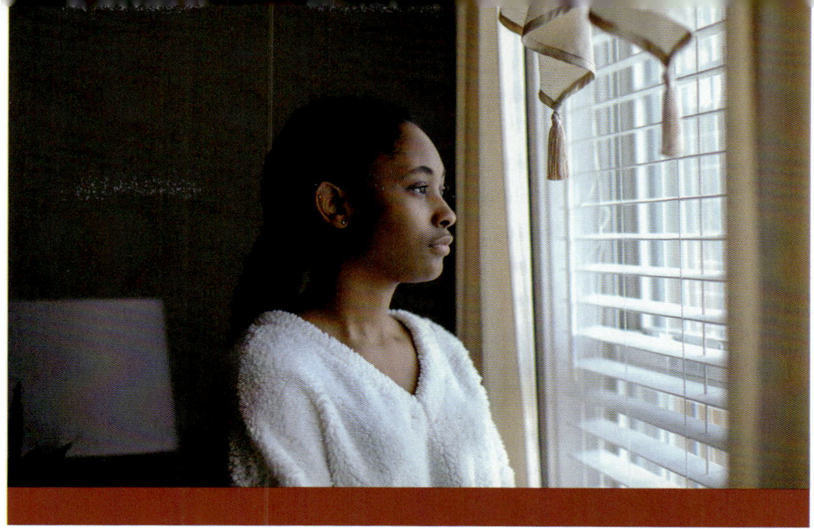

Some phobias can make it difficult to leave the home and interact with others.

to get disability benefits. These benefits are monthly payments. They are given to low-income people with disabilities.

People with phobias may face these and other challenges. But mental health professionals can help. All phobias can be treated. Isaac Marks is a professor and mental health expert. He says, "People can overcome phobias."[9]

HOW ARE PHOBIAS TREATED?

The first step to treatment is diagnosis. Certain mental health professionals can make diagnoses. These include psychologists and therapists. **Psychiatrists** are trained to do this too. Doctors are often involved as well. They look at the patient's physical health. Other things

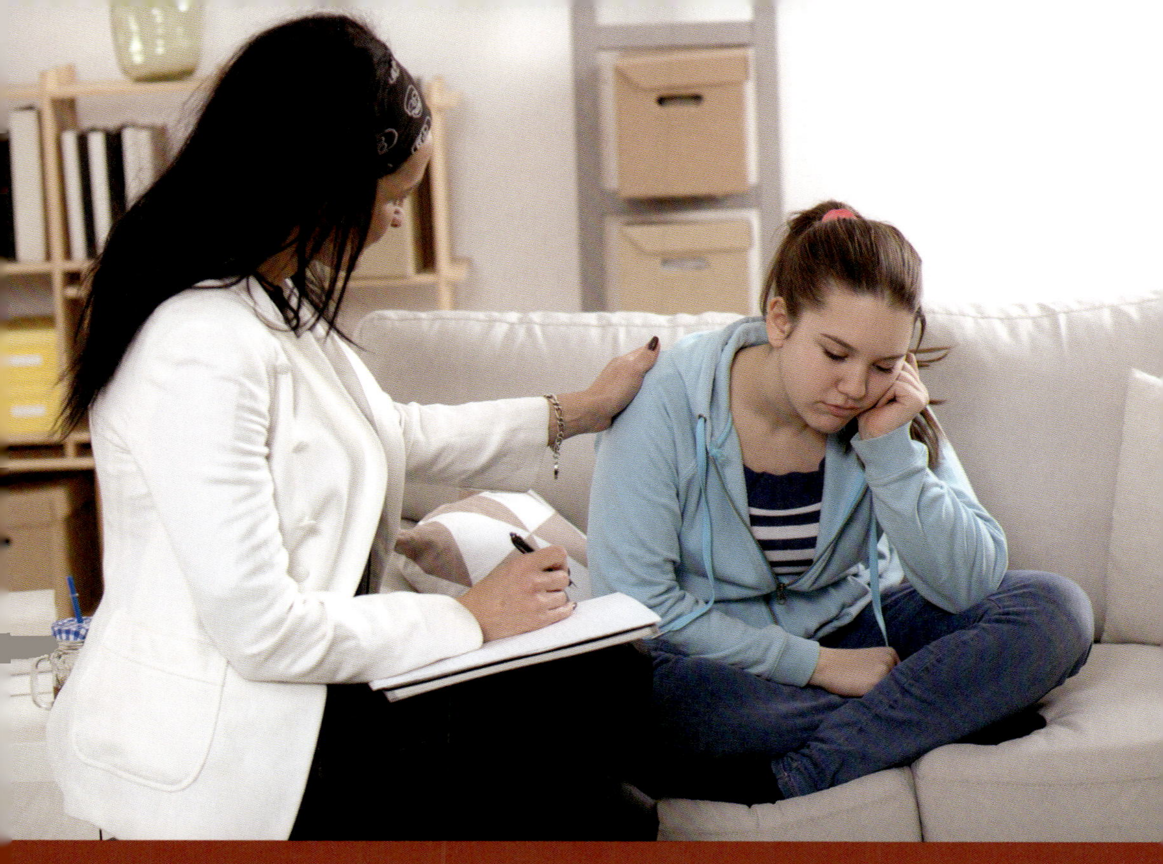

Mental health professionals are able to diagnose phobias.

could be causing a patient's anxiety. Some

substances may cause anxiety. These

include caffeine and alcohol. Anxiety

can also be a side effect of medications.

Some medical conditions can cause

anxiety too. These include certain heart and brain diseases. The symptoms may look similar to phobias.

THERAPY

After a diagnosis, people can begin therapy. Therapists provide this treatment. Therapists include counselors or social workers. They help people learn how to manage their phobias. They also help people set and achieve goals. For example, someone with SAD might want to make a friend. The therapist helps him figure out how to do this.

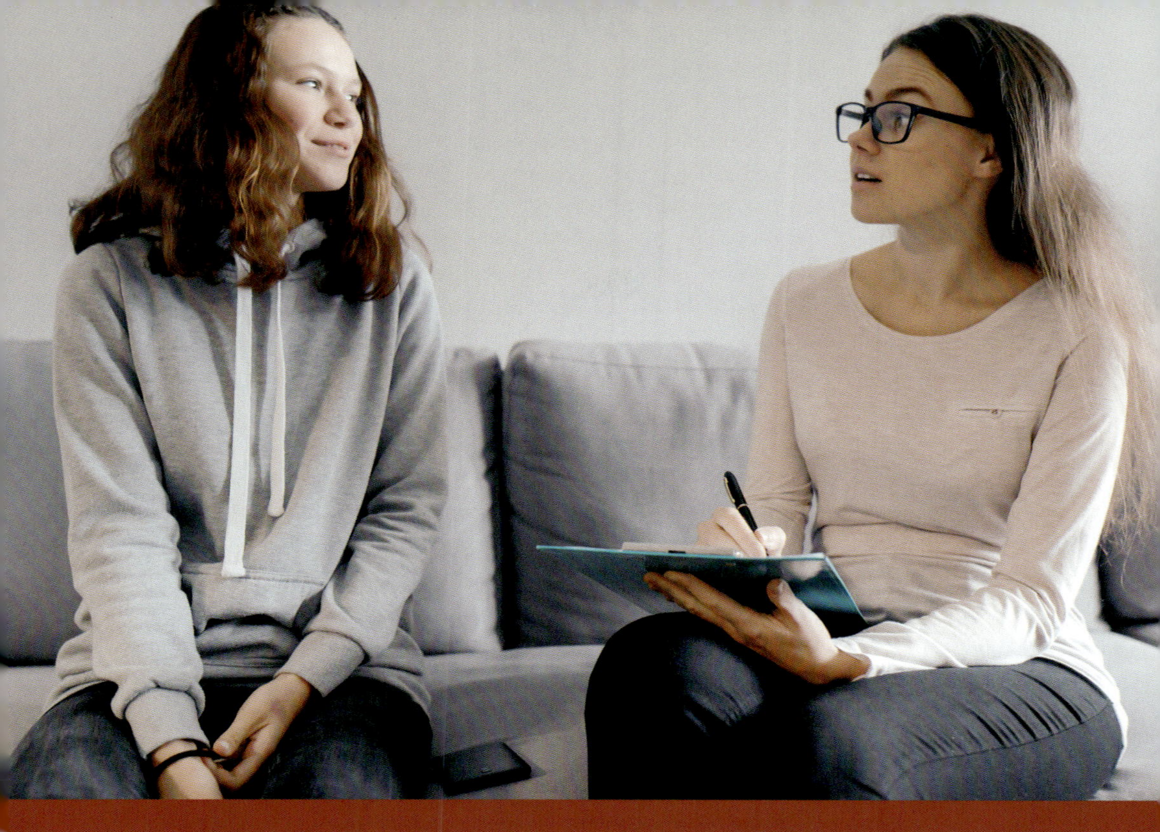

Therapy can help someone manage her phobia.

Cognitive behavioral therapy (CBT) is often used to treat phobias. People explore their thoughts and feelings about triggers. They learn how their thoughts influence their behaviors. For example, CBT can be used to treat a person with a dog phobia.

Certain thoughts and feelings are triggered

when the person sees a dog. The person

might think, "That dog will attack me!"

This thought adds to her feeling of fear.

Then she chooses how to act. Because she

CULTURAL DIFFERENCES

There are many cultural groups in the United States. Some phobias are more common in certain cultural groups. For example, people may worry about offending others. They fear they will make others uncomfortable. This fear is most common in Japanese and Korean cultures. People with this fear might have SAD symptoms. They may be diagnosed with SAD.

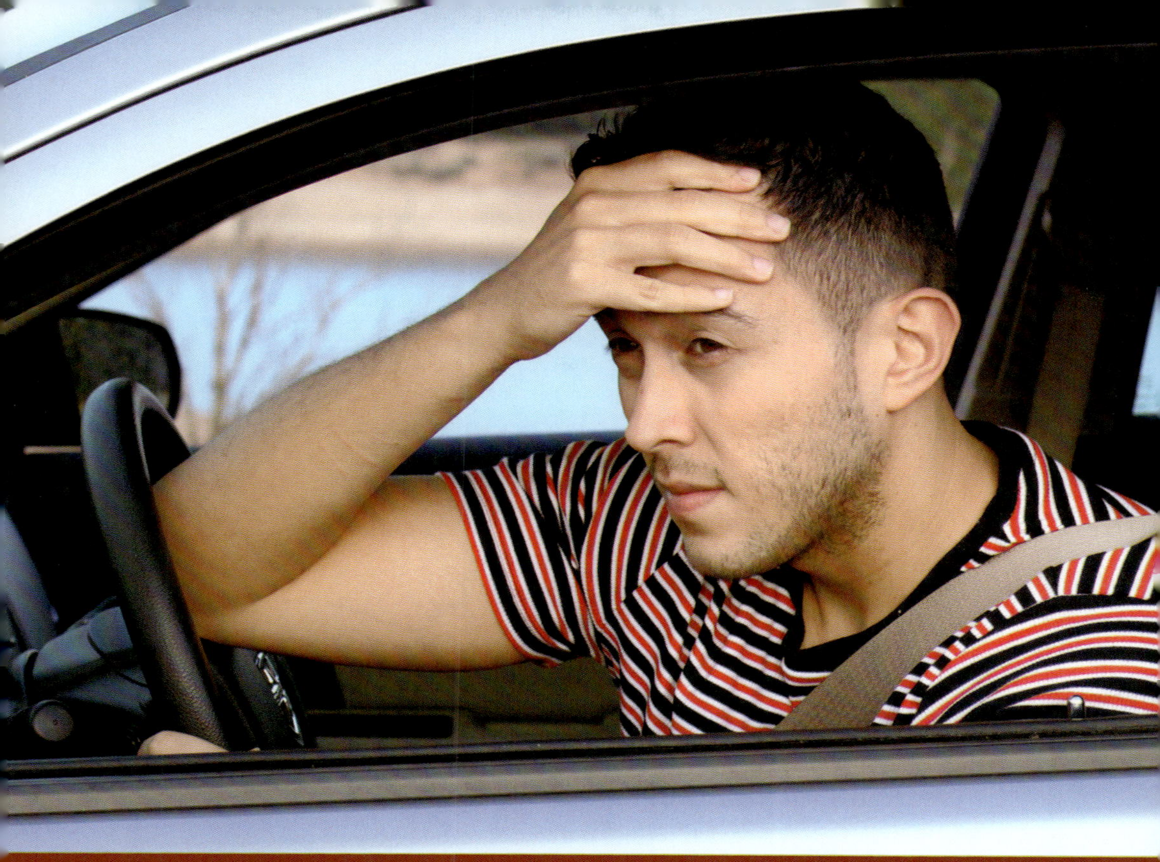

is scared, she may run away. Running away

becomes a habit.

CBT teaches people to recognize these

patterns. People learn to challenge their

negative thoughts. The person with the dog

phobia could learn to change her thoughts.

Her first thought might be that all dogs

are dangerous. But she could challenge

this. She could tell herself that no one

would have dogs as pets if they were all

dangerous. Then she might be less fearful.

Over time, her behavior might change. She

might stop avoiding dogs.

FACING FEARS

Exposure therapy can also help people with

phobias. This approach is part of CBT. The

first step is to make a list of triggers. For

example, someone with a dental phobia has

specific triggers. These might include the

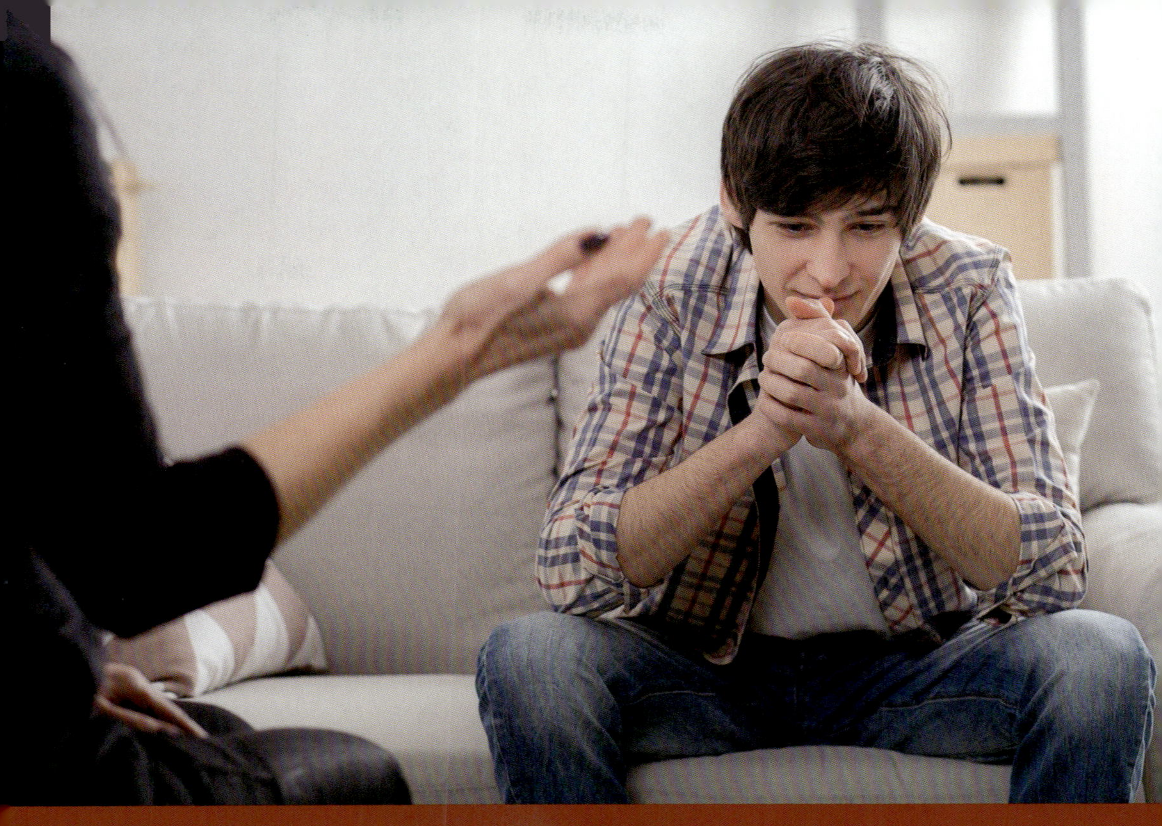

Therapists and patients work together to create a plan for exposure therapy.

sound of a dental drill. Thinking about going

to the dentist could also cause anxiety.

The person puts these triggers on his list.

He orders them from least to most fearful.

Next, the therapist teaches relaxation

skills. These skills might include singing.

Another skill is muscle relaxation. The

person then faces his fears. He starts with

the situation that is the least fearful. This

might be thinking about going to the dentist.

He does relaxation exercises. He repeats

this process. He gradually moves on to

more fearful situations. For example, the

therapist may play the sound of a dental

drill. The patient learns to manage his

anxiety during these situations. The process

is similar for treating SAD or agoraphobia.

Someone with agoraphobia might think

about a public place. Someone with

SAD might think about a social situation.

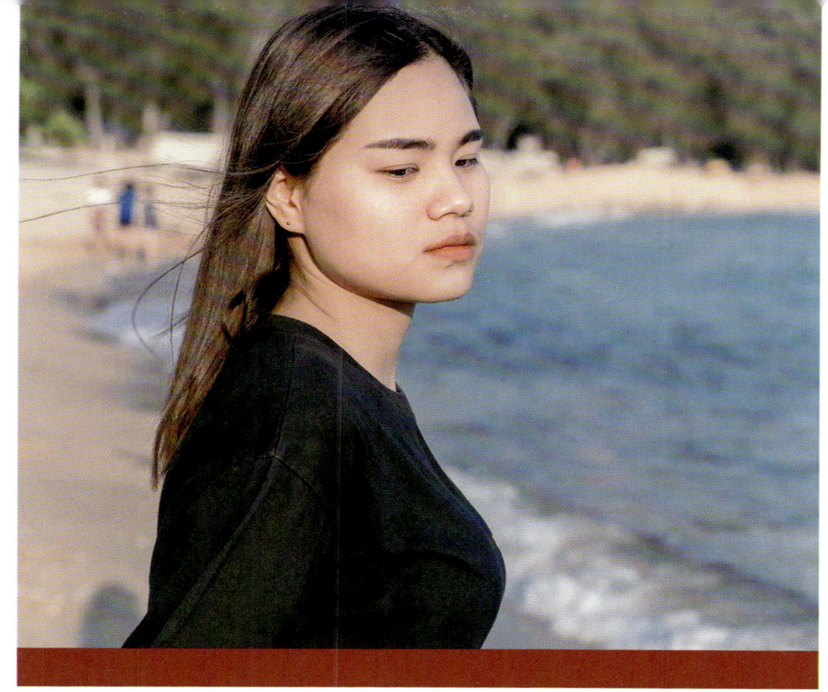

Someone with a fear of water gradually learns to face her fear with exposure therapy.

Dr. Craig April treats phobias using exposure therapy. He says, "You've got [to] face [your fear] to get past it. There's really no other way. . . . The challenge is in facing that fear gradually."[10]

After imagining their triggers, people might look at pictures next. Finally, they may face these triggers in real life. Therapists guide them through this process. Ellen O'Connell Whittet has a snake phobia. She went through exposure therapy. She started by imagining snakes. Then she looked at photos of them. She had to view the photos

JOE McCAULEY'S STORY

Joe McCauley had a water phobia. His phobia started when he was twelve years old. He was in a scuba diving class. There was a problem with his scuba gear. McCauley's diving partner accidentally cut off his oxygen trying to fix it. McCauley finally faced his fear after more than twenty-five years. In 2014, he signed up for a swim race in the Pacific Ocean. The race was 2 miles (3 km) long. McCauley finished the swim. He had learned to manage his fear.

from a few feet away at first. Her next

goal is to see a snake in real life. She pays

attention to her anxiety level. She says, "I

decide how far to push myself, and when

I've had enough for the day."[11] This gives her

a sense of control over her phobia.

People with phobias may learn other

skills in therapy too. Someone with SAD

may learn social skills. These skills might

include eye contact. The person might

practice giving speeches.

Therapy is the best treatment for

phobias. Medication can also help. Doctors

and psychiatrists **prescribe** medication.

It can help people cope with a specific event. For example, someone with SAD might take medication before giving a speech. Medication treats the person's symptoms. It reduces anxiety. Doctors help people find the right medication. They make sure patients understand how much medicine they should take.

COPING SKILLS

People can develop skills outside of therapy. These skills can help them manage their anxiety. Journaling can help people understand their phobias. It can help them

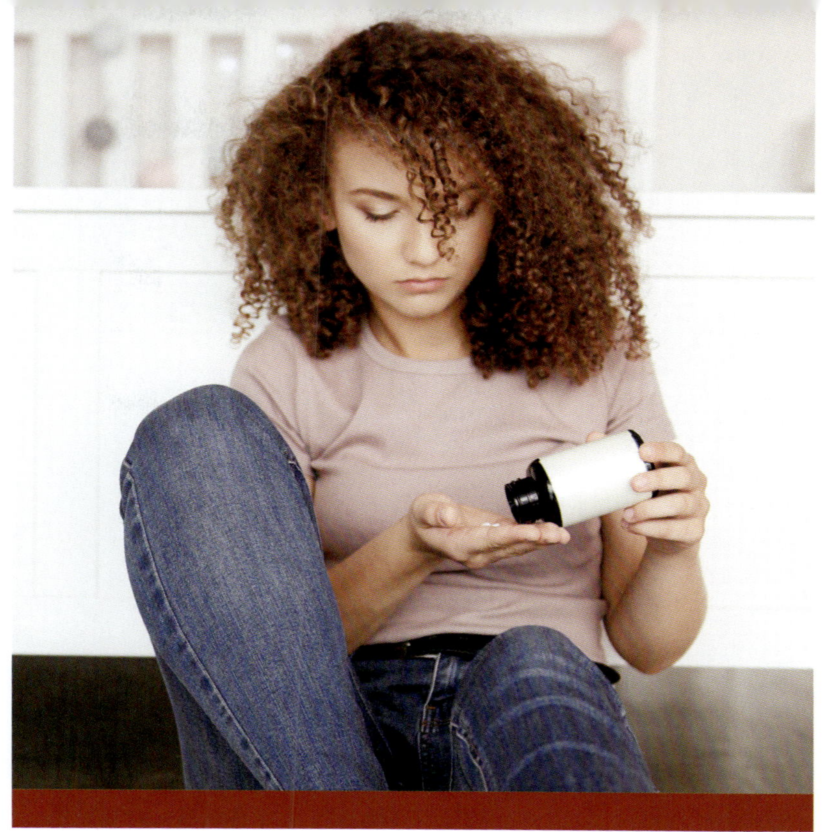

A patient may take medication to help treat her phobia.

identify their thoughts and feelings. This skill

can pair well with CBT.

Relaxation exercises may also help.

These might include yoga and meditation.

Meditation is a quiet activity. People focus

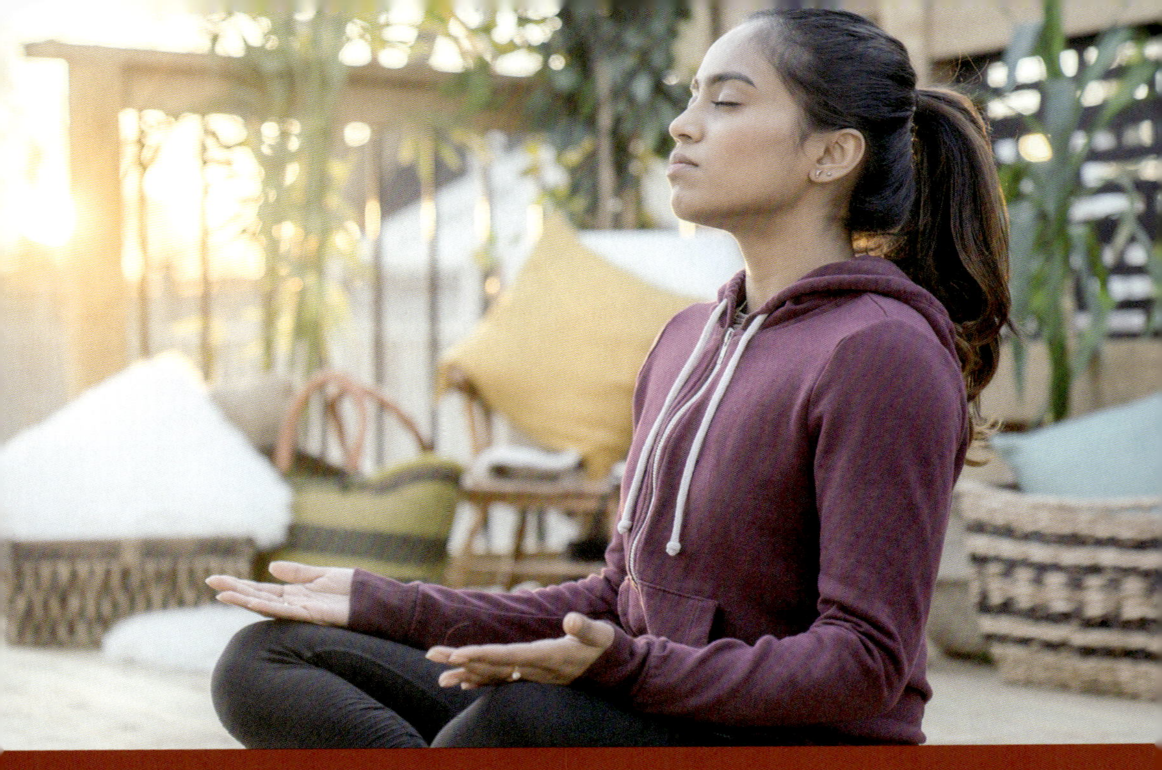

Meditation is a coping skill that can help with managing anxiety.

on their breathing. People notice their

thoughts and feelings. But they do not

get caught up in them. This process can

reduce anxiety.

People can also join support

groups. They talk to people with similar

experiences. They also talk about their coping skills. Others in the group help people with phobias feel less alone. Reaching out to others is an important coping skill.

It can be hard to ask for help. But it is rewarding. Phobias are treatable. People with phobias can work with therapists and learn to manage their anxiety. They can lead full lives. Ellie has agoraphobia. She struggled with this phobia for years. Then she sought therapy. It helped her face her fear. She says, "I have found myself again."[12]

GLOSSARY

blood pressure
the force of blood as it moves through a person's body

discrimination
the act of treating someone differently based on his or her race or other characteristics

genes
information within a person's cells that can be passed down in families and determines traits such as eye color

hormones
chemicals released within a person's body that help the body grow and develop

LGBTQ
lesbian, gay, bisexual, transgender, or queer/questioning

prescribe
to write a prescription, which is an official recommendation that tells someone which medication to take

psychiatrists
doctors who treat mental, emotional, or behavioral disorders

stigma
a societal attitude about something that creates shame around it and makes people feel embarrassed to be associated with it

symptoms
thoughts, behaviors, or actions that show a person has a disorder

trigger
to cause or bring about an intense, negative emotion

SOURCE NOTES

CHAPTER ONE: WHAT ARE PHOBIAS?

1. Aimee Browes, "Living with Claustrophobia: 'I'm Too Afraid to Lock My Bathroom Door,'" *BBC*, January 16, 2019. www.bbc.co.uk.

2. Stacey Griffith, "How I Overcame My Fear of the Ocean After Nearly Drowning," *Time*, May 22, 2017. www.time.com.

3. Quoted in "Phobia, Anxiety and OCD Interviews," *April Center for Anxiety Attack Management*, n.d. www.kickfear.com.

4. Agata Boxe, "Afraid of Needles? You May Want to Blame Your Genes," *Discover*, September 10, 2019. www.discovermagazine.com.

CHAPTER TWO: HOW DO PHOBIAS AFFECT PEOPLE?

5. "Marie's Story—Agoraphobia," *WayAhead Mental Health Association*, n.d. https://understandinganxiety.wayahead.org.au.

6. Quoted in Ranit Mishori, "No, No, Not the Needle!" *Washington Post*, April 13, 2004. www.washingtonpost.com.

CHAPTER THREE: HOW DO PHOBIAS AFFECT SOCIETY?

7. Quoted in Melissa Dittmann, "When Health Fears Hurt Health," *American Psychological Association*, July/August 2005. www.apa.org.

8. Quoted in Mishori, "No, No, Not the Needle!"

9. Quoted in "Coping with Fears and Phobias," *NHS Inform*, February 5, 2021. www.nhsinform.scot.

CHAPTER FOUR: HOW ARE PHOBIAS TREATED?

10. Quoted in "Phobia, Anxiety and OCD Interviews."

11. Ellen O'Connell Whittet, "I Developed a Snake Phobia After My Sexual Assault," *Allure*, July 11, 2017. www.allure.com.

12. "Escaping My Agoraphobia," *Mind*, July 9, 2018. www.mind.org.uk.

FOR FURTHER RESEARCH

BOOKS

Heidi Ayarbe, *Living witn Phobias*. San Diego, CA: ReferencePoint Press, 2019.

Alexis Burling, *Understanding Panic Attacks*. San Diego, CA: BrightPoint Press, 2021.

Therese M. Shea, *What Are Phobias?* New York: Rosen, 2021.

INTERNET SOURCES

"Anxiety: When You Are Worrying About Things," *Women's and Children's Health Network*, June 28, 2018. www.cyh.com.

"Fears and Phobias," *KidsHealth*, n.d. www.kidshealth.org.

"Specific Phobia Basics," *Child Mind Institute*, 2021. https://childmind.org.

WEBSITES

Anxiety and Depression Association of America (ADAA)
www.adaa.org

The ADAA shares information about depression and anxiety disorders such as phobias. It also helps people find treatment.

Mental Health America (MHA)
www.mhanational.org

MHA raises awareness of disorders such as phobias. It also supports research and laws to help people with mental health issues.

National Alliance on Mental Illness (NAMI)
www.nami.org

NAMI educates people about mental health issues including phobias and anxiety disorders. It offers resources and information. NAMI also has a helpline. People can call this phone number for support.

IMAGE CREDITS

ABOUT THE AUTHOR

Maddie Spalding is an author and mental health advocate. She has written books on a variety of topics. She lives and works in Minneapolis, Minnesota.